CHUBBY TO HEALTHY

STRATEGIC WAY TO ACHIEVE WEIGHT LOSS

MAXWELL STONE

DISCLAIMER

This book is only intended to provide knowledge that is relevant to daily life. Every effort has been made to provide accurate, current, trustworthy, and comprehensive information. In no way should you take this as medical advice; instead, you should speak with your physician.

TABLE OF CONTENTS

INTRODUCTION

Being solid is highly wanted by all individuals. Sickness and infirmity are not just collected by some coincidence; large numbers of the determinants of well-being are notable. We know from research that infirmity as well as most ongoing or longstanding illnesses are connected with undesirable ways of life, for instance, smoking, wrong eating regimen, actual latency, and overstated liquor utilization. Today, we allude to these circumstances as "government assistance or way of life sicknesses." Individuals learn ways of behaving and propensities as opposed to those being intrinsic and these ways of behaving and propensities can be impacted by one's own solidarity and be supplanted by other more well-being-supporting ones. Nonetheless, it isn't generally as basic as it sounds to transform one's way of life, since it is usually grounded in an underlying condition. The point of this book was to introduce a portrayal of how individuals themselves, to an impressive degree, can influence their well-being in a positive heading by taking on a wellbeing advancing way of life.

CHAPTER 1

WAYS TO DETERMINE MACRONUTRIENTS FOR WEIGHT REDUCTION.

What are Macronutrients?
Macronutrients (or macros for short) are the particular particles that contain energy and supplements to make up calories. Each calorie of food that you eat can be separated into three principal bunches that contain energy (calories). The quality and measure of macronutrients you consume consistently decide your body synthesis and your presentation. Which are;
CARBOHYDRATE
PROTEIN
FATS
ALCOHOL
Your body separates macronutrients and utilizes their supplement thickness to make energy, fabricate the body fundamentally, make synthetic responses, and invigorate the sound working and arrival of chemicals. What you eat can decidedly or adversely

influence how you feel, play out, your mindset and, surprisingly, your behaviour. However, micronutrients themselves don't contain calories. Just the macros (protein, fat, carb, and liquor) yield calories.

Sugars (1g carb = 4 calories)
Protein (1g Protein = 4 calories)
Fats (1g Fat = 9 calories)
Liquor (1g liquor = 7 calories)
You unquestionably can follow calories, yet if you're searching for a more precise way to deal with working on your general well-being, body structure, and execution, you will need to follow your macros. When contrasted with following calories, which ignores what the calories come from (protein, carb, fat), following macros guarantees that the calories you eat are getting you the planned outcomes.

Step-by-step instructions to Decide on Macros Deciding the macros on a nourishment name is straightforward. Investigate a sustenance name and separate it, beginning with the serving size. Frequently, items contain 2-4 servings in a bundle (or more) so it's significant your serving size matches the macros that you log. Try not to get found out in the thoughtless customer trap, feeling that you're consuming short of what you are.

How To Track Your Macros?

The most effective method to follow your macros is tradable with how to count your macros and it's actually very basic and straightforward:

Read nourishment labels

Utilize a food scale or estimating cups as opposed to eyeballing

Log your admission on a portion of food following application or in a diary

By doing these three stages, you can all the more likely see exactly the number of calories that are in food varieties and that you're placing into your body to be more mindful of how they impact your body arrangement, energy levels, and execution.

What number of Macros Do I Really want?

How much macros (protein, carbs, fat) you want consistently are subject to your own objectives. Is it safe to say that you are hoping to get fitter, lose muscle-to-fat ratio, increment bulk/size, keep up with weight, work on general well-being and health, and so forth.? Without knowing the objective, there truly is no straightforward reply to this inquiry.

What Is The Best Macronutrient Proportion?
The best macronutrient proportion is the one that...
works for yourself as well as your body. Each
individual is different in their requirements, body
creation, hereditary cosmetics, and generally
speaking well-being, which is the reason working
1:1 with a sustenance mentor can be very useful.
Besides the fact that they keep you responsible and
on target, they assist with showing you your singular
body and what levels and kinds of supplements fuel
it best so that you're not simply making efforts in
that frame of mind with your proportions.

That being said, you're not confused, we guarantee.
To decide the number of macros you need, you want
to lay out a macronutrient proportion for your body
and your objectives.

A general macronutrient proportion for adjusted
nourishment is:

45-60% starches
20-35% fats
30-45% protein

Contingent upon the objective, you will either increment or abate the rates inside the gatherings. The most effective method to Compute Your Macros

Since it has become so obvious what macronutrients are, the number of calories they have, and a general macronutrient proportion for adjusted well-being (and a couple of general objectives), you can start to compute your macros (by doing some math). While the macronutrient proportion is written in rates, the sustenance data found on a name or in a piece of food is given in grams.

This is the thing you should be aware of before ascertaining your macros:
The number of calories that you eat in a day (generally, we'll involve 2300 calories for instance)
Decide your optimal proportion of protein, carbs, and fat (we'll utilize half carbs, 25% protein, and 25% fat for instance)
Increase your everyday calories by your rates
Partition your calorie aggregates by their calorie-per-gram number.

CHAPTER 2

WAYS TO DETERMINE CALORIES FOR WEIGHT REDUCTION:

To get in shape, you want to eat fewer calories than you consume. In principle, this sounds straightforward. Be that as it may, calorie counting is one method for handling this issue.

What Are Calories?
Calories are a proportion of energy, ordinarily used to gauge the energy content of food sources and refreshments.

A dietary calorie is characterized as how much energy is expected to raise the temperature of 1 kilogram of water by 1 degree Celsius.

You utilize the calories that you eat and drink for fundamental capabilities like breathing and thinking, as well as everyday exercises like strolling, talking and eating.

Any excess calories you eat will be put away as fat, and reliably eating more than you consume will cause weight gain over time. It's very normal to hear that calories don't make any difference and that calorie counting is an exercise in futility.

Nonetheless, concerning your weight, calories do count.

This is a reality that has been demonstrated endlessly and time again in logical tests called an overloading review.

These examinations ask individuals to gorge and hence measure the effect on their weight and well-being intentionally.

All overloading investigations have discovered that, when individuals eat a bigger number of calories than they copy off, they put on weight.

This straightforward truth implies that counting calories and restricting your intake can be successful to forestall weight gain or get in shape, as long as you figure out how to adhere to it.

The number of calories you need relies upon factors like orientation, age, weight and activity level.

For instance, a 25-year-old male competitor will require a larger number of calories than a 70-year-elderly person who doesn't work out.

The following are 5 hints to counting calories:

Be ready: Before you start, get a calorie counting application or online instrument, conclude how you will quantify or gauge partitions and make a dinner arrangement.

Peruse food marks: Food names contain heaps of valuable data for calorie counting. Ensure you check the part size suggested on the bundle.

Eliminate enticement: Dispose of the unhealthy food in your home. This will assist you with picking better bites and make it more straightforward to hit your objectives.

Go for the gold, weight reduction: Don't cut calories excessively low. Although you'll get fit quicker, you might feel terrible and be less inclined to adhere to your arrangement.

Fuel your activity: The best health improvement plans incorporate both eating routine and exercise. Make a point to eat to the point of still having the energy to work out.
Be that as it may, concerning weight reduction, calories do count.

Even though it sometimes falls short for everybody, you might observe that counting calories is a compelling method for shedding pounds and keeping them off.

CHAPTER 3

WAYS TO SLOW DOWN SUGAR WEIGHT GAIN.

Eating an excess of sugar might be decimating your well-being.

Added sugar, which is the sugar tracked down in soft drinks, desserts, and other handled food sources, has been displayed to add to heftiness, type 2 diabetes, coronary illness, malignant growth, and tooth rot.

The research proposes that most Americans eat somewhere in the range of 55-92 grams of added sugar every day, which is identical to 13-22 teaspoons of table sugar every day addressing around 12-16% of day-to-day calorie consumption.

This is altogether more than the Dietary Rules for Americans' suggestion of getting under 10% of your everyday calories from added sugars.

In any case, cutting added sugars from your diet can be a challenge. Here are ways of preventing weight gain from sugar.

1. Cut back on sweet beverages:
Most added sugars in the American eating routine come from sweet drinks, sodas, sports drinks, caffeinated drinks, improved teas, and others.

Also, drinks that many individuals see as solid, like smoothies and organic product juices, can in any case contain bewildering measures of added sugar.

For instance, 1 cup (271 grams) of cranberry juice mixed drink contains more than 7 teaspoons of sugar (31 grams).

Also, your body doesn't perceive calories from drinks similarly to those from food. Calories from drinks are consumed rapidly, bringing about a quick expansion in your glucose level.

Drinks likewise don't cause you to feel as full as strong food, so individuals who polish off heaps of calories from drinks don't eat less to redress. Lessening your admission of sweet beverages can assist with weight reduction and work on generally speaking well-being.

Here are some better refreshment choices that are normally low in sugar:

water
unsweetened shimmering water
homegrown teas

dark or green tea
espresso.

2 . Stay away from sweet treats:
Most pastries don't give a lot of in that frame of
mind of health benefit. They're stacked with sugar,
which causes glucose spikes that can leave you
feeling drained and hungry and cause you to pine for
more sugar.

Grain and dairy-based treats, like cakes, pies,
doughnuts, and frozen yoghurt, represent over 18%
of the admission of added sugar in the American
eating regimen.

Assuming you need something lower in added sugar
that can in any case fulfil your sweet tooth, attempt
these other options:

new natural product
Greek yoghurt with cinnamon or natural product
prepared organic products with cream
dull chocolate (70% cocoa or higher)
A reward for eating an entirely natural product?
Trading sugar-weighty treats for new or prepared
natural products decrease your sugar admission as

well as expands the fibre, nutrients, minerals, and cell reinforcements in your eating regimen.

 3. Avoid sauces with added sugar:
Sauces like ketchup, grill sauce, spaghetti sauce, and sweet stew sauce are typical in many kitchens. Be that as it may, a great many people don't know about their sugar content.

A 1-tablespoon (17-gram) serving of ketchup contains around 1 teaspoon (5 grams) of sugar. That implies ketchup is an incredible 29% sugar, sweeter than frozen yoghurt.

Search for fixings and sauces marked "no additional sugar" to scale back the secret sugars in these items.

Different choices for preparing your food that is normally low in addcd sugars incorporate spices and flavours, bean stew, mustard, vinegar, pesto, mayonnaise, and lemon or lime juice.

4. Eat entire food varieties
Entire food varieties haven't been handled or refined. They are additionally liberated from added substances and other fake substances. These food

sources incorporate entire natural products, vegetables, entire grains, vegetables, and meat on the bone.

At the opposite finish of the range are super-handled food sources. These are arranged food varieties that contain salt, sugar, fat, and added substances in blends that are designed to taste astounding — which makes it hard to direct your admission of these food varieties.

Instances of super-handled food sources are soda pops, sweet grains, chips, and cheap food.

Practically 90% of the added sugars in the normal American's eating routine come from super-handled food sources, while just 8.7% come from food varieties arranged without any preparation at home utilizing entire food sources.

Attempt to cook without any preparation whenever the situation allows, so you can stay away from added sugars. You don't need to prepare elaborate dinners. Basic arrangements like marinated meats and cooked vegetables will give you heavenly outcomes.

5. Check for sugar in canned food varieties:
Canned food varieties can be a helpful and economical option to your eating routine, yet they can likewise contain a great deal of added sugar.

Leafy foods contain normally happening sugars. Be that as it may, these aren't normally an issue since they don't influence your glucose the same way added sugar does.

Keep away from canned food varieties that are pressed in syrup or have sugar on the fixing list. Natural products are adequately sweet, so go for variants marked "stuffed in water" or "no additional sugar."

Assuming you purchase canned natural products or vegetables that do have added sugar, you can eliminate some of it by flushing them in water before you eat them

6. Be cautious with "sound" handled nibble food sources:
Some handled nibble food sources have a "well-being corona." They appear to be solid from the get-go, and words like "healthy" or "regular" might be

utilized in their showcasing to cause them to appear to be more grounded than they are.

Shockingly, these bites (for example, granola bars, protein bars, and dried organic products) can contain the same amount of sugar as chocolate and pieces of candy.

Dried organic products are an incredible model. It's brimming with fibre, supplements, and cancer-prevention agents. Notwithstanding, it likewise contains concentrated measures of regular sugar (and a few renditions might be "candy-coated" with extra added sugar), so you ought to direct your admission to hold back from going overboard.

Here are some sound low-sugar nibble thoughts:

nuts and seeds
no-sugar-added jerky
hard-bubbled eggs
new organic product.

7. Read marks:
Eating less sugar isn't so natural as staying away from sweet food varieties. You've previously seen

that it can be concealed in improbable food varieties like ketchup and granola.

Luckily, food makers are presently expected to reveal included sugars and food names. You'll see added sugars recorded under all-out starches on food sources that contain them.

On the other hand, you can check the fixing list for sugar. The higher on the fixing list sugar shows up, the more sugar the thing contains since fixings are recorded from the most elevated add up to the least sum utilized by weight.

8. Consider eating more protein:
High sugar consumption has been connected to expanded hunger and weight gain. On the other hand, an eating routine low in added sugar but high in protein and fibre might make the contrary difference, decreasing craving and advancing completion.

Protein has additionally been displayed to diminish food desires straightforwardly. One investigation discovered that rising protein in the eating routine by 25% decreased desires by 60%.

To check sugar desires, stock up on protein-rich entire food varieties, like meat, fish, eggs, full-fat dairy items, avocados, and nuts.

9. Switch to regular zero-calorie sugars:
There are a few fake sugars available that are thoroughly liberated from sugar and calories, for example, sucralose and aspartame.

In any case, these counterfeit sugars might be connected to lopsided characteristics in stomach microbes that can prompt less fortunate glucose control, expanded food desires, and weight gain. Therefore, it could be ideal to stay away from counterfeit sugars as well.

A few other regular zero-calories sugars show a guarantee. These incorporate stevia, erythritol, priest natural product, and allulose.

They are normally inferred, although they do go through some handling before they show up at your neighbourhood supermarket. In any case, research on these sugar choices is continuous.

10. Limit things with high sugar content in the house:
Assuming you keep high-sugar food varieties in the house, you might be bound to eat them. It takes a great deal of self-control to stop yourself on the off chance that you just need to go similarly to the storage room or refrigerator to get a sugar hit.

Be that as it may if you live with others it tends to be difficult to keep specific food sources out of the house — so you might need to have an arrangement set up for when sugar desires to strike. Studies have shown that interruptions, for example, doing puzzles, can be extremely powerful at decreasing desires.

If that doesn't work, then attempt to keep some solid low-sugar snacks in the house to chomp on all things being equal.

11. Get enough rest:
Great rest propensities are inconceivably significant for your well-being. Unfortunate rest has been connected to sadness, unfortunate fixation, decreased safe capability, and corpulence.

Nonetheless, the absence of rest may likewise influence the sorts of food you eat, inclining you toward decisions that are higher in sugar, fat, salt, and calories.

One investigation discovered that individuals who hit the hay late and didn't get an entire night's rest devoured more calories, cheap food, and pop and fewer products of the soil than the people who hit the sack before and got an entire night's rest.

Furthermore, a new observational review noticed that higher admissions of added sugar were related to an expanded gamble of a sleeping disorder in postmenopausal ladies.

Assuming that you're battling to quit settling on high-sugar food decisions, getting better rest might assist you with recapturing some control.

CHAPTER 4

HAVING A SOLID MOTIVATED SOUL.

Numerous things can disrupt everything while attempting to carry on with a sound way of life. Our timetables can be loaded with responsibilities that make it hard to make a customary everyday practice, like working long moves or around evening time, examining while likewise having some work, or adjusting to having kids and working or considering. No matter what the reasons you may be finding it challenging to keep a sound way of life, there are little changes you can make to assist with spurring yourself to remain solid.

6 methods for getting persuaded to carry on with a sound way of life
1. Be positive towards yourself
If you have gone some time without practising or eating steadily, this is alright and you shouldn't regret or blame yourself. No matter what your ongoing way of life is, you can make new propensities and roll out sure improvements for your

prosperity. It is so vital to Have positive self-conviction. Have faith in your capacity to change your well-being propensities or some other parts of your way of life you need to.

2. Put forth objectives

Laying out your sensible objectives is an incredible method for keeping yourself propelled to remain solid. On the off chance that, for instance, you might want to start or return to working out, defining yourself an objective of what you might want to accomplish inside a specific time can assist with keeping you on target. An objective could be something like being dynamic a specific number of times in seven days or joining a sporting group activity or exercise class.

Instances of objective setting can be:

Strolling 5000 stages per day

3. Roll out little improvements to better choices additional time

It might appear hard to adhere to a solid eating routine if you need to change your ongoing eating regimen and eating designs totally. All things being equal, if you need to pursue better decisions, begin little and pick one change to what you eat day to day, so it is more sensible. For instance, on the off chance that you assume you are eating an excess of handled food sources or meat, decide to transform one of your dinners daily to something more plant-based.

Keep in mind, getting in shape ought not to be the essential focal point of changing to a better eating routine. A better spotlight may be on the general advantages that having a fair eating routine can have on your body and brain.

4. Practice the way that suits you
It tends to be difficult to remain propelled to practice assuming you believe you have no time or you loathe it. There are a lot of ways that you can squeeze practice into your everyday daily schedule without forfeiting accomplishing something you appreciate. Rolling out little improvements, for example, strolling or cycling a piece of your drive, practising on your mid-day break or while heating the pot can assist you with fitting practice in any event when you don't think you have the opportunity.

5. Practice with another person

Practising with someone else can be an effective method for remaining spurred, as you can push each other to in any case practice on days you may not feel like you need to. At the point when you practice with another person you can likewise challenge each other to drive yourselves that smidgen further each time. Going to practice classes can likewise be an incredible method for remaining inspired as you can feel part of a local area while working out and having some good times.

6. Get sufficient rest

Getting no less than 8 hours of rest a night can assist with keeping you inspired over the day as you will have more energy to do what means quite a bit to you. By consolidating rest, with a decent eating regimen and exercise your body will have more energy. Expanded energy levels can assist with keeping you propelled to lead a sound way of life, and in different parts of your life. It merits an opportunity to focus on yourself. Driving a solid way of life can assist with working on your mindset, fixation, emotional well-being and by and large prosperity.

CHAPTER 5

MAKING TIME/PLAN FOR EXERCISE.

If you truly have any desire to get results through the scale and keep on gaining ground after some time, you want to focus on working no less than four to five days out of each week. However, recall that you'll move toward this. To begin, you could believe you should do a few days of the week and move gradually up to five days. The three parts of an even workout routine incorporate vigorous exercise, strength preparation, and adaptability training. Start by arranging more modest exercise meetings. Start with 5 brief meetings daily and step by step move gradually as long as 30-moment or even extended meetings. With a workout, each meeting counts. Having 3-4 20-minute exercises seven days a week rather than a solitary 2-hour session is better.

Begin with dynamic extending. The principal thing
to do is warm up. ...
Pick your objective regions. Picking a section to
zero in on assists provide you with better guidance
in your everyday practice. ...
Settle on the numbers. ...
End on the cardio. ...
Cool down and do some formative stretches.

CHAPTER 6

STEP BY STEP INSTRUCTIONS to CONTROL DISTRESS AND ACHING.

Deferred beginning muscle touchiness is a regular
cycle that demonstrates your muscles are getting
more grounded, so there's no risk in braving it. Yet,
it tends to be uncomfortable. Fortunately, there are a
couple of things you can do to assist with facilitating
the aggravation.

The following are seven ways to alleviate sore muscles:

1. Get moving. In all honesty, one of the most amazing ways of lessening muscle irritation is to get them rolling. You can hit the treadmill or dynamic recuperation, which incorporates extending, froth rolling or yoga.

2. Be sure to heat up. A significant piece of safeguarding your muscles is ensuring they're prepared for use before you challenge them. Set aside a few minutes for a few minutes of warm-up before each exercise.

3. Progress gradually into another activity program. Going from 0 to 60 doesn't help your muscles. Allowing them to adjust can assist with restricting the seriousness of your irritation. While beginning another exercise routine daily practice or while increasing the power, simply make certain to do so sluggishly throughout a few days or weeks.

4. Soak in a salt shower. Absorbing warm water with Epsom salts can assist with loosening up your muscles and alleviate torment.

5. Take a painkiller. This won't accelerate the muscle-recuperating process, yet it can assist you with tolerating the distress related to it.

6. Try a split-day schedule. Assuming you like to work out each day, consider dividing your exercises by muscle bunch. For example, one day is legs and the following is arms. This will assist with guaranteeing that you're giving each muscle bunch sufficient opportunity to recuperate before you train it once more.

CHAPTER 7

FOLLOWING UP ON YOUR DEVELOPMENT

Weight reduction can be seen around the belly and laps first. This is because your body stores fat in

various areas. For example, men hold more fat around their midsection, while ladies store it on their thighs and hips. Weight reduction steadily begins with a decrease in midsection size. Within three to a half years, an individual can see a 25 to 100 percent improvement in their solid wellness.
 Here are a few elements to show that you're moving in a decent course:

1. You're not voracious continually
Accepting for the time being that you're shedding fats since you changed your eating routine to integrate more proteins and fewer carbs and fat, you could see that you feel full faster. That is because the amino acids in dietary protein convey a fulfilment message to your cerebrum — and that sign isn't sent by eating a similar number of calories in fat or carbs.

2. Your feeling of prosperity gets to the next level

 Individuals who were attempting to shed fats announced that they felt greater essentialness, more discretion, less sorrow, and less tension than they had felt before their weight reduction.

On the off chance that you're not feeling these profound advantages yet, don't surrender: Study members didn't report these upgrades at the half-year point. Large mental changes appeared at the year interviews.

3. Your garments fit in an unexpected way
You might see that you don't need to leap to pull on your pants, even before you see a major distinction on the scale — which can rouse you to continue doing what you're doing.
 Around 77% of ladies and 36 per cent of men said they're persuaded to shed pounds to further develop how their garments fit their bodies.

4. You're seeing some muscle definition
It can require some investment — normally weeks or months — to develop fortitude and see muscle definition. How quickly you see changes will rely upon your body and the sort of activity you've integrated into your arrangement.

Young ladies constructed more bulk in their legs when they performed more reiterations of leg twists

and presses with a lighter burden than with fewer
reps and a heavier burden.

5. Your body estimations are evolving
A good reduced size is good news for your general
well-being. Studies show that 430 individuals in a 2-
year weight in the board program noticed that a
decrease in midsection estimation was related to
further developed results in pulse, glucose, and
cholesterol.

Studies have drawn an immediate connection
between your midsection periphery and your gamble
of cardiovascular illness. Whether the scale
expresses you're down, a looser belt implies better
heart well-being.

6. Your constant aggravation moves along
Weight reduction can assist with diminishing agony,
particularly in the weight-bearing region of the
body, similar to the lower legs and lower back.

 Individuals who lost no less than 10% of their body
weight saw the best improvement in ongoing agony
around weight-bearing zones.

Losing 20% of body weight decisively further developed knee torment and irritation in individuals with joint pain.

7. You're going to the washroom more — or less — habitually
Changing what you eat may influence your solid discharge designs.

Killing meat and adding more salad greens and vegetables to your eating routine can further develop blockage while adding more creature protein to your eating regimen (as numerous paleo and keto counts calories do) can make certain individuals more inclined to stop.

If you're worried about the distinctions in your defecations, or on the other hand on the off chance that they're obstructing your efficiency, it very well might be smart to talk with a nutritionist or medical care supplier about tweaking your arrangement to further develop your stomach wellbeing.

8. Your pulse is descending

Too much fat can adversely affect your pulse, making you weak against strokes and respiratory failures

One method for cutting down your pulse is to shed pounds with a better eating regimen and greater development. Assuming that you're getting fitter, you're lessening the stress on your heart and starting to standardize your circulatory strain

9. You wheeze less
Wheezing has a convoluted relationship with weight. Individuals (particularly ladies) who have metabolic conditions (a forerunner to diabetes) tend to wheeze.

Wheezing and dozing may try and cause weight gain. Hence, weight reduction is many times one of the designated treatments for individuals who wheeze and who have resting messes.10. Your state of mind improves
Putting out strong improvements to your diet can bring a good state of mind and more energy.

CHAPTER 8

PAY SPECIAL ATTENTION TO CHANGE.

The main phase of weight reduction is the point at which you will generally lose the most weight and start to see changes in your appearance and how your garments fit. It typically occurs within the initial 4 months and a half. The greater part of the weight reduction in this stage comes from carb stores, protein, and water — and less significantly, body fat. Altogether, it can take somewhere in the range of a multi-week to a while to see observable weight reduction results. Everything relies upon your day-to-day activity level, your activities, and the amount you eat every day.
You have Quite a lot more ENERGY.
Your neighbourhood café has seen a drop in deals since you never again depend on various coffees to work.
Individuals come to you for weight reduction exhortation.

That's right — it's your chance to give out exhortations on the significance of fitting in 10,000 everyday advances, chugging water and learning segment control. Be glad that individuals are admiring you!

You'll carry on with a more drawn-out, better life. Can we just look at things objectively, weight reduction isn't just about squeezing into your thin pants — that is only the cherry on top of realizing that you'll be around for your friends and family from here onward, indefinite.